From Plate to Peak: Achieve Your Fitness Goals with the Right Diet

Norman M. Jackson

Table of contents

INTRODUCTION

Understanding the Role of Nutrition in Fitness

Nutrition plays a pivotal part in getting optimal fitness levels and general health. Within the world of fitness, the importance of nutrition cannot be overstated, as it serves as the base upon which physical success and well-being are built. Understanding the complex link between dietary choices and exercise achievements is crucial for anyone trying to reach their peak physical potential.

Essentially, nutrition serves as the fuel that drives the body, giving the energy necessary for various physical tasks. Carbohydrates, for instance, act as the main energy source, providing the body with easily available fuel for quick use during workouts. Proteins, on the other hand, play a vital part in muscle repair and growth, helping in the recovery process after hard exercise. Additionally, fats add to hormone control and serve as a concentrated source of energy, especially during endurance activities.

A thorough understanding of the importance of nutrient timing and makeup is crucial in improving workout performance. Pre-workout nutrition impacts energy levels and stamina, while post-workout meals affect muscle recovery and growth. The careful balance of macronutrients and micronutrients in the diet directly affects not only physical performance but also general health and well-being.

Furthermore, hydration is an often overlooked yet critical part of nutrition in exercise. Adequate water intake ensures proper bodily processes and helps control body temperature during exercise, thus avoiding dehydration and its negative effects on performance.

Beyond the physical factors, the role of nutrition in promoting mental clarity and attention cannot be ignored. A well-balanced diet rich in important vitamins and minerals supports brain function, helping in keeping focus during workouts and promoting a positive attitude suitable to achieving fitness goals.

In summary, comprehending the intricate interplay between nutrition and exercise is important for anyone wanting to improve their physical performance and general health. By understanding the effect of different nutrients on the body's processes, individuals can make informed food choices that support their exercise efforts and contribute to a healthy and sustainable lifestyle.

CHAPTER I: Setting the Foundation

Creating a balanced and lasting diet plan includes adding a range of nutrient-rich foods into your daily meals. This includes a mix of whole grains such as brown rice, quinoa, and whole wheat pasta, along with an assortment of fresh fruits and veggies like spinach, berries, and bell peppers. Lean protein sources like chicken, fish, and tofu serve as important components, while healthy fats from avocados, nuts, and olive oil provide crucial energy and support for bodily processes.

Managing portion amounts plays a key part in keeping a well-balanced diet. For instance, a balanced breakfast might consist of a palm-sized piece of lean protein, a fist-sized serving of complex carbohydrates, and a large portion of leafy greens or coloured veggies. Understanding the value of portion control helps avoid overeating and supports weight management goals.

Moreover, comprehending the importance of meal timing can improve the body's metabolic processes and energy consumption. Eating regular meals throughout the day, including a nutritious breakfast to restart the metabolism, and adding healthy snacks in between meals can help keep stable energy levels and avoid unhealthy cravings. Additionally, being aware of post-workout diet by eating a mix of carbs and protein aids in muscle repair and refills energy stores.

By combining these examples into a daily dietary routine, people can create a strong nutritional base that not only supports their exercise goals but also promotes general well-being and long-term health.

CHAPTER 1i: Building a Balanced and Sustainable Diet Plan

Constructing a dietary plan that smoothly blends nutritional balance with environmental sustainability lays the groundwork for long-term health and happiness. This chapter digs into the basic concept of adding nutrient-dense whole foods, such as bright fruits, leafy veggies, whole grains brimming with fibre, and lean meats drawn from organic and socially raised sources. By stressing the consumption of these wholesome, unprocessed foods, individuals can fortify their bodies with important vitamins, minerals, and antioxidants, boosting their immune system and supporting vital bodily processes.

Moreover, supporting sustainability through dietary choices is important for fostering an environmentally aware approach to nutrition. Encouraging the selection of locally sourced food, this chapter shows the reduction of carbon impact and helps local farming communities. By minimising the consumption of highly processed and packaged foods, people can contribute to the decrease of trash and support sustainable food production practices, thus playing a part in saving the planet's natural resources for future generations.

In addition to the focus on whole foods, this chapter also argues for the concept of balance. It underscores the significance of mindful eating, emphasising the importance of amount control and the consumption of meals in a calm and attentive way. By encouraging people to enjoy each bite, pay attention to hunger cues, and respect the body's signs of fullness, this method creates a good relationship with food. It pushes people to foster a greater understanding of their dietary needs and preferences, allowing for a sustainable eating pattern that supports general well-being and avoids the development of unhealthy eating habits.

By adopting these strategies, individuals can lay the basis for a balanced and sustainable diet that not only nurtures their personal health but also adds to the preservation of the environment, creating a holistic approach to wellness that benefits both people and the world.

CHAPTER 2: Fueling Your Performance

Diving into the complex link between diet and sports performance, this chapter reveals the key strategies for improving physical output in both strength training and endurance exercises. With a primary focus on the significance of macronutrient balance, the chapter emphasises the role of carbohydrates in providing readily available energy for high-intensity workouts, proteins in supporting muscle repair and growth, and fats in contributing to sustained energy during prolonged activities.

Understanding the value of hydration in sports success is also a core theme of this chapter. Highlighting the critical role of water in regulating body temperature, lubricating joints, and transporting nutrients, the chapter emphasises the need for consistent hydration before, during, and after exercise to maintain optimal physical function and prevent the adverse effects of dehydration on performance.

Furthermore, the chapter dives into the nuances of pre- and post-workout nutrition, elucidating the significance of eating suitable meals or snacks to improve performance and aid in efficient muscle repair. It emphasises the need for a mix of carbohydrates and proteins before a workout to provide sustained energy and support muscle function, while post-workout meals rich in protein and carbohydrates aid in replenishing glycogen stores and supporting muscle repair and growth.

By providing practical insights and evidence-based recommendations on how to fuel the body effectively for different types of physical activities, this chapter equips athletes and fitness enthusiasts with the knowledge to fine-tune their diets and optimise their nutritional intake for enhanced physical performance. Understanding the complex link between nutrition and athletic efforts is key to unlocking one's full potential and reaching top performance in the chase of fitness goals.

CHAPTER 2i: Optimising Nutrition for Strength and Endurance

Within the world of athletic performance, the need for specialised nutrition to respond to the demands of both strength-based training and endurance exercises is important. This chapter digs into the specific dietary details needed to support and improve muscle strength, healing, and growth, as well as the important nutritional strategies aimed at boosting endurance and sustaining energy levels during longer workouts.

For strength training, the focus lies on consuming appropriate amounts of high-quality proteins to enable muscle repair and growth. This includes adding lean forms of protein such as chicken, fish, and plant-based alternatives into the diet. Additionally, the chapter shows the importance of complex carbohydrates in providing a continuous release of energy, supporting intense weight lifting workouts, and promoting muscle glycogen replenishment for optimal recovery.

Conversely, when handling endurance activities, the focus changes towards ensuring a sufficient amount of easily digestible carbs to power prolonged physical effort. Incorporating sources like whole grains, fruits, and starchy veggies aids in keeping glycogen stores, preventing the start of tiredness, and sustaining energy levels throughout longer cardio workouts. Moreover, the chapter underscores the importance of adding healthy fats, such as those found in nuts, seeds, and avocados, which serve as a supplementary source of energy during long endurance workouts.

Furthermore, the chapter dives into the significance of meal timing and the consumption of healthy pre- and post-workout meals. Highlighting the necessity of consuming a combination of carbohydrates and proteins before engaging in strength-based exercises to optimise performance and muscle recovery, it also emphasises the importance of consuming easily digestible carbohydrates during endurance activities to maintain energy levels and stave off muscle fatigue.

By providing practical insights into the tailored nutritional needs of both strength and endurance activities, this chapter equips athletes and fitness enthusiasts with the knowledge required to customise their diets, ensuring optimal performance and sustained energy levels during various types of physical exertion. Understanding the specific dietary needs for strength and endurance lays the groundwork for achieving top performance and improving fitness goals in both areas.

CHAPTER 3: The Power of Supplements

In the goal of better sports performance and general health, the utilisation of dietary supplements has gained broad attention. This chapter looks into the varied role of supplements in complementing and optimising nutritional diet to support exercise goals and promote general health.

One of the key main points of the chapter revolves around understanding the possible benefits and limits of different types of supplements. It elucidates the role of important vitamins such as vitamin C, which aids in immune function and tissue repair, and vitamin D, crucial for bone health and muscle function. Additionally, the chapter discusses the importance of minerals like iron, essential for oxygen movement and red blood cell production, and calcium, vital for bone strength and muscle contraction. By emphasising the role of these key micronutrients, the chapter underscores their input to general physical well-being and athletic success.

Furthermore, the chapter explores the possible benefits of supplementing with specific compounds such as omega-3 fatty acids, famous for their anti-inflammatory qualities and support for cardiovascular health. It also looks into the role of protein supplements in helping muscle repair and growth, especially in cases where dietary protein intake may be insufficient. Moreover, the talk stretches to the possible benefits of certain herbal products and their effect on boosting energy levels, promoting healing, and lowering exercise-related inflammation.

However, the chapter also shows the importance of exercising care when incorporating supplements into one's diet. It stresses the necessity of contacting healthcare professionals or qualified nutritionists to ensure the safe and effective use of supplements, as well as to avoid possible harmful effects or combinations with current medicines.

By providing guidance on selecting reputable supplement brands, understanding proper dosage recommendations, and emphasising the importance of quality assurance and regulation in the supplement industry, this chapter empowers individuals to make informed decisions regarding the incorporation of supplements into their dietary regimen. By leveraging the power of supplements effectively and carefully, individuals can boost their nutritional intake and support their fitness efforts, leading to improved performance, enhanced healing, and general well-being.

CHAPTER 3i: Enhancing Your Diet for Maximum Results

Achieving ideal results in terms of health and fitness hangs on the adoption of an effective and useful dietary approach. This chapter digs into the multiple strategies aimed at maximising the benefits gained from one's diet, stressing the integration of nutrient-dense foods and the careful use of supplementation to support individual health and fitness goals.

A significant focus of the chapter swirls around the addition of nutrient-dense foods, such as a wide variety of fruits, vegetables, whole grains, and lean sources of protein. Emphasising the importance of a diverse and varied diet, the chapter underscores the role of these whole foods in providing important vitamins, minerals, antioxidants, and dietary fibre necessary for promoting general well-being and supporting various body functions.

Furthermore, the chapter discusses the possible role of targeted supplementation in bridging nutritional gaps and improving specific health and exercise goals. It examines the potential benefits of incorporating supplements such as multivitamins to ensure comprehensive micronutrient intake, as well as the use of specialised supplements like protein powders or amino acids to support muscle repair and growth in the context of rigorous training or exercise regimes.

In addition to promoting the merging of nutrient-dense foods and supplements, the chapter stresses the importance of unique nutritional changes. It recognizes the importance of tailoring dietary plans to meet specific health and exercise needs, taking into account factors such as personal goals, dietary tastes, and any underlying health considerations. By pushing for a personalised approach to nutrition, the chapter encourages people to develop a deeper knowledge of their dietary needs and to make informed choices that match with their unique goals.

Moreover, the chapter shows the value of keeping consistency and balance in dietary practices to achieve sustainable and long-lasting effects. It stresses the importance of fostering healthy eating habits and supporting mindful consumption, encouraging people to create a positive relationship with food and to view dietary changes as a sustainable lifestyle choice rather than a temporary fix.

By equipping individuals with comprehensive insights into the integration of nutrient-dense foods, the strategic use of supplements, and the significance of personalised dietary adjustments, this chapter empowers individuals to enhance their diets for maximum results, fostering improved overall well-being and bolstered performance in their pursuit of health and fitness goals.

CHAPTER 4: Navigating Challenges

Embarking on a dietary journey often offers numerous challenges that can hinder progress and longevity. This chapter digs into the varied world of dietary obstacles, offering practical insights and effective strategies for beating these hurdles and developing a resilient approach to nutrition.

A core theme of the chapter swirls around managing cravings and beating temptations that may derail one's dietary efforts. It stresses the importance of developing mindfulness and self-awareness to identify triggers that lead to unhealthy eating habits. By supporting the adoption of mindful eating practices and encouraging the discovery of healthier alternatives to meet cravings, the chapter equips individuals to develop a more balanced and controlled approach to controlling their dietary desires.

Additionally, the chapter discusses the challenges posed by lifestyle changes and the necessity of changing food habits to fit with growing circumstances. It stresses the significance of setting realistic and doable goals, fostering steady lifestyle changes, and finding social support to foster responsibility and drive. By acknowledging the dynamic nature of life and the need for change in dietary methods, the chapter urges people to welcome adaptability as a key component of long-term dietary success.

Furthermore, the chapter navigates the complexities associated with different dietary restrictions and tastes, providing practical advice on how to meet specific nutritional needs while keeping a well-balanced and enjoyable diet. Whether handling food allergies, intolerances, or lifestyle-based dietary choices, the chapter argues for the study of diverse culinary options and the incorporation of creative cooking techniques to ensure a satisfying and nutritionally adequate dietary experience.

Moreover, the chapter emphasises the importance of building a good and sustainable relationship with food, supporting the idea of food as nourishment and pleasure rather than a source of restriction or deprivation. By fostering a holistic understanding of the psychological and emotional aspects of dietary habits, the chapter encourages people to value self-care and self-compassion in their dietary journey, fostering a resilient attitude that supports long-term success and general well-being.

By providing comprehensive insights into navigating various challenges encountered on the dietary path, this chapter aims to empower individuals to overcome obstacles, cultivate resilience, and foster a positive and sustainable approach to nutrition, ultimately facilitating long-term success in their pursuit of health and wellness.

CHAPTER 4 I:

Overcoming Dietary Obstacles and Maintaining Long-Term Success

The path to keeping a healthy and balanced diet is often filled with hurdles that can test even the most determined individuals. This chapter digs into the intricate world of dietary challenges, offering complete insights and effective strategies for overcoming these hurdles and developing a sustainable approach to nutrition that leads to long-term success and general well-being.

One of the primary hurdles people often face is the challenge of handling cravings and dealing with temptations that can derail their dietary efforts. This chapter emphasises the importance of understanding the psychological and physiological factors driving cravings and urges, encouraging readers to develop awareness methods that allow them to spot triggers and control impulses more effectively. By exploring healthier options and encouraging a better knowledge of the root causes of cravings, individuals can develop a more balanced and controlled approach to controlling their food impulses, eventually leading to healthier long-term habits.

In addition to controlling cravings, the chapter discusses the major challenge of keeping lifestyle changes necessary for having a healthy diet. It admits the difficulty of fitting dietary changes into one's daily routine, especially in the face of demanding schedules and competing goals. The chapter shows the importance of setting realistic and achievable goals, supporting gradual lifestyle changes, and finding social support to promote responsibility and motivation. By arguing for the merging of small, sustainable changes over time, the chapter encourages people to view dietary modifications as a gradual and adaptive process, supporting long-term adherence and success.

Furthermore, the chapter navigates the difficulties associated with different dietary restrictions and tastes, addressing the unique challenges faced by people with specific nutritional needs. Whether addressing food allergies, intolerances, or lifestyle-based dietary choices such as vegetarianism or veganism, the chapter advocates for the exploration of diverse culinary options and the incorporation of creative cooking techniques to ensure a satisfying and nutritionally adequate dietary experience. It provides practical tips for meal planning, recipe swaps, and managing social settings, enabling people to accept their dietary choices while keeping a balanced and satisfying diet that supports their long-term health and well-being.

Moreover, the chapter emphasises the importance of creating a positive and lasting relationship with food, encouraging people to view food as fuel and pleasure rather than a source of restriction or lack. It handles the emotional and psychological aspects of dietary habits, stressing the need for self-compassion and self-care in the face of failures or difficulties. By supporting a holistic approach to nutrition that spans both physical and mental well-being, the chapter empowers individuals to foster resilience and develop a healthy mindset that supports long-term success and satisfaction in their dietary journey.

By providing thorough insights and practical strategies for overcoming dietary obstacles, this chapter serves as a valuable resource for individuals looking to develop sustainable and resilient dietary habits, eventually leading to long-term success and improved overall health and wellness.

CONCLUSION

Sustaining Your Fitness Journey Through a Holistic Approach to Nutrition and Wellness

Maintaining a consistent and successful fitness journey requires a holistic approach that includes not only physical exercise but also a thorough knowledge of nutrition and general health. This chapter digs into the critical role of a well-rounded and sustainable dietary plan in supporting long-term fitness goals, while also stressing the importance of combining overall health practices that feed the mind, body, and spirit. By exploring the interconnections between nutrition, exercise, mental well-being, and self-care, the chapter aims to encourage people to maintain their fitness journey through a balanced and thorough approach to general health and wellness.

At the core of this overall approach is the understanding that diet plays a key role in fueling the body and supporting physical performance. The chapter stresses the importance of consuming a varied diet that includes a wide range of nutrient-dense foods, including fruits, veggies, whole grains, lean proteins, and healthy fats. By providing important vitamins, minerals, and antioxidants, these foods help improve body processes, support muscle growth and healing, and enhance general well-being. The chapter further discusses the significance of proper hydration, stressing the critical role of water in keeping optimal physical performance and supporting the body's natural detoxification processes.

Beyond nutrition, the chapter argues for the merging of holistic health practices that support mental and social well-being. It shows the benefits of incorporating mindfulness methods, such as meditation and deep breathing exercises, to reduce stress, improve focus, and increase general cognitive function. Furthermore, the chapter supports the adoption of regular physical activities beyond structured exercise routines, such as yoga, Pilates, or nature walks, to promote flexibility, balance, and general physical and mental resilience.

Additionally, the chapter underscores the importance of proper rest and healing in sustaining a successful fitness journey. It dives into the importance of quality sleep in supporting muscle repair, hormone control, and general immune function. By highlighting the effect of sleep on both physical and mental well-being, the chapter encourages individuals to prioritize creating regular and restful sleep habits as an integral part of their general wellness practice.

Moreover, the chapter explores the role of self-care in creating a positive and sustainable attitude. It argues for the practice of self-compassion, encouraging individuals to value activities that bring joy, rest, and satisfaction. By creating a healthy lifestyle that includes time for relaxation, hobbies, and social ties, individuals can maintain a sense of general well-being and satisfaction, thereby supporting their drive and commitment to their fitness journey.

By providing thorough insights into the integration of nutrition, holistic health practices, and self-care, this chapter serves as a useful guide for individuals looking to develop a sustainable and well-rounded approach to their fitness journey. By recognizing the interconnected nature of physical, mental, and emotional well-being, people can foster a complete understanding of their general health and wellness, thus sustaining their commitment to long-term fitness success and better quality of life.